Nursing Care Plan

Volume 1: Arthritis, Alzheimer's disease, Diabetes Mellitus, Hypertension, AIDS and Pneumonia

Solomon Barroa, R.N.

Copyright 2013

All rights reserved. No part of this book may be reproduced by any means, electronic, mechanical, photocopying, recording, scanning or otherwise without permission from the author. The author reserves the right not to be responsible for the correctness, completeness or quality of the information provided. Liability claims regarding damage caused by the use of any information provided, including any kind of information that is incomplete or incorrect, will be rejected. The information contained in this book does not constitute medical advice, and is for information and educational purposes only. Consult your health care provider regarding health concerns.

To Dr. Lee Robbins, Mary Ann, Rosario, Vicente, Benedicto, and Robert.

Introduction and Purpose

Nursing is always associated with caring and interventions. This is been taught in school and is consistent in professional work. Nursing professionalism is projected through the nurse's knowledge, skills and personality in caring for the sick person. However much professional work done by the nurse, is not simply an automatic process. The nurse utilizes the method called the nursing process and then formulates nursing care plan based on the problems of the client.

The care plan is formally written and is created in coordination with the different members of the healthcare team. The nursing process begins with the assessment of the problem. Data is gathered and a nursing diagnosis formed. Setting goals comes next followed by the interventions to accomplished the goals that have been set. The final step involves evaluating the interventions and modifying them if the goal has not been met.

This book is intended and prepared for both student nurses and nurse professionals. It aims to provide direction for nursing care plans related to the diseases and conditions commonly encountered. It also serves as a quick reference guide for making a care plan thereby saving time and effort at the work place. Depending on the existing policies of facilities and agencies, nursing care plans may differ slightly. As nursing evolves, so do the nursing care plans.

The author does not intend this text to substitute for the existing knowledge of the reader. The intention is to provide educational material that can be used as a reference in formulating a care plan. The author believes that the reader has his or her own unique ability in formulating a suitable nursing care plan. The correctness of the materials in this book is based upon the rigorous method and usage of research materials. The author does not claim any responsibility in relation to the correctness and usability of the information presented in this book. Reader's discretion is advised and warranted in using any type of information in this book.

For inquiries, the author can be reached at:

solomon_barroa@yahoo.com

or at the link :

http://www.amazon.com/Solomon-Barroa-RN/e/B00AV3V34S

Table Of Contents

Chapter 1 The Nursing Process — 7

Chapter 2 Nursing Care Plans for Arthritis — 8

Nursing Care Plan 1 — *10*
Nursing Diagnosis # 1 — *10*
Nursing Care Plan 2 — *11*
Nursing Diagnosis # 2 — *11*
Nursing Care Plan 3 — *12*
Nursing Diagnosis # 3 — *12*

Chapter 3 Nursing Care Plans for Alzheimer's Disease — 13

Nursing Care Plan # 1 — *14*
Nursing Diagnosis # 1 — *14*
Nursing Care Plan # 2 — *15*
Nursing Diagnosis # 2 — *15*
Nursing Care Plan # 3 — *16*
Nursing Diagnosis # 3 — *16*

Chapter 4 Nursing Care Plans for Diabetes Mellitus — 17

Nursing Care Plan # 1 — *20*
Nursing Diagnosis # 1 — *20*
Nursing Care Plan # 2 — *21*
Nursing Diagnosis # 2 — *21*
Nursing Care Plan # 3 — *22*
Nursing Diagnosis # 3 — *22*

Chapter 5 Nursing Care Plans for Hypertension — 23

Nursing Care Plan # 1 — *24*
Nursing Diagnosis # 1 — *24*
Nursing Care Plan # 2 — *25*
Nursing Diagnosis # 2 — *25*
Nursing Care Plan # 3 — *26*
Nursing Diagnosis # 3 — *26*

Chapter 6 Nursing Care Plans for AIDS — 27

Nursing Care Plan # 1 — *28*
Nursing Diagnosis # 1 — *28*
Nursing Care Plan # 2 — *29*

Nursing Diagnosis # 2	*29*
Nursing Care Plan # 3	*30*
Nursing Diagnosis # 3	*30*

Chapter 7 Nursing Care Plans for Pneumonia   31

Nursing Care Plan # 1	*32*
Nursing Diagnosis # 1	*32*
Nursing Care Plan # 2	*33*
Nursing Diagnosis # 2	*33*
Nursing Care Plan # 3	*34*
Nursing Diagnosis # 3	*34*

References   35

Index   36

Chapter 1 The Nursing Process

Nursing is a profession that cares for and assists clients in transitioning from a disease process to the period of recovery. It is dynamic and has evolved through the decades. The delivery of nursing care requires a nursing care plan formulated whenever a problem arises. The problems occur in response to the disease process. A nursing care plan is formulated by the nurse utilizing the nursing process. The nursing process is the systematic resolution of a patient's health problem comprising assessment, diagnoses, planning, implementation and evaluation.

Assessment is the systematic and dynamic collection, validation and communication of a client's information or data. It is accomplished through activities such as data gathering, confirmation and comparison, systematic organization, analyses and documentation of the data.

There are 2 types of data: subjective and objective. Subjective data are descriptions coming from the patient regarding experiences such as pain and dizziness. Objective data involves data that are observable and measurable such as edema and redness and laboratory findings. There are common sources of data; primary and secondary. Primary data involves collection directly from the patient whereas secondary data does not involve the patient and is obtained from such sources as medical records, laboratory results and other people.

Diagnosing is a process that utilizes the standardized nursing diagnosis. The purpose of diagnosing is to identify health care needs. Nursing diagnosis is a statement of a patient's health problems based on analyzed data.

Nursing diagnosis follows the format of identifying the problem, causes and the signs and symptoms. Planning is the process of determining the goals of care and courses of action to be performed. It involves setting priorities, goals and planning nursing care.

Goals are characterized as SMART (specific, measurable, attainable, realistic and time framed). Implementing is the process of putting the plan into action. It involves skills in cognition, communication and intervention abilities.

There are 3 common types of nursing actions; independent, interdependent and dependent. Independent nursing actions arises from the nurses themselves, interdependent nursing action arises from collaborating with other members of the healthcare team, and dependent nursing actions arise from the instructions and prescriptions of a physician. Evaluating is a process of measuring the extent to which the specified goals in the planning phase of the nursing process are achieved. It involves analyzing results and the patient's health attainments.

Chapter 2 Nursing Care Plans for Arthritis

Arthritis is defined as the inflammation of the joints. The inflammation is due to different factors such as the degenerative changes that occur in the structures within the joints. Swelling occurs due to the body's response to the changes and in turn causes compression of nerves and releases prostaglandin inducing a painful sensation. The nursing care plan for a client with arthritis will focus on existing problems such as pain, loss of ability to move the affected joint, deformity, weakness and fatigue and among others.

Osteoarthritis is a condition where there is gradual degeneration and degradation of the cartilage within the joints. Osteoarthritis commonly affects the fingers, hips, feet, spine and knees. Over time due to aging and use, the cartilage degenerates. The elastic cartilage that serves as a cushion between the bones gradually deteriorates and breaks apart causing the bone ends to rub on each other and develop uneven outgrowths and spurs called osteophytes. Joint cartilage becomes fissured, synovial fluid leaks out of the subchondral bone and cysts develop. Research has shown that osteoarthritis more commonly occurs in men over 45 and women over 55 years of age.

The common causes of osteoarthritis include rheumatoid arthritis which, while itself often an autoimmune disease, can in turn lead to osteoarthritis; arteriosclerosis; obesity; trauma and family history. The degenerative changes produce symptoms such as joint stiffness, pain aggravated by movement, crepitus (cracking noises) upon movement, muscle spasm and loss of ability to move the joint. There is also weight loss, fever, contractures and coldness of the extremities. Bony enlargements called Heberden's nodes or Bouchard's nodes develop. Heberden's nodes occur near the fingertips while Bouchard's nodes occur at the middle of the fingers.

Osteoarthritis is commonly diagnosed through x-rays. The result of the x-ray will show narrowing of joint spaces as well as bony outgrowths around the joint. Early conservative treatment consists of analgesics such as acetaminophen and moderate exercises for the affected part. It is believed that exercises preserve the functionality of the affected joint, strengthens the muscles to reduce stress on the joint as well as reduces the painful sensation. Exercises are supervised and guided by healthcare professionals to avoid pressure and stress on the joint. Symptomatic management includes application of heat to reduce stiffness or spasm and cold to reduce swelling and pain, elevation of extremities to reduce swelling and utilization of assistive devices to reduce weight bearing on the affected extremities. Arthroscopy and arthroplasty may be performed. Arthroscopy is the insertion of a viewing tube to smooth and repair the cartilage. Arthroplasty is the total replacement of the joint. Injection of corticosteroid into the joint is also prescribed in cases of severe pain.

Rheumatoid Arthritis is an autoimmune disorder affecting the tissues and organs of the body causing systemic inflammation. It particularly attacks the synovial (movable) joints. The synovium (capsule around a joint) becomes swollen and fibrous tissue develops. The inflammation causes destruction of the cartilage and ankylosis (fusion) of the joints. Synovitis with edema causes the proliferation of different blood materials that leads to the destruction and fibrosis of the cartilage (fibrous ankylosis) as well as calcification of fibrous tissue (osseus ankylosis). Aside from affecting the synovial joints, rheumatoid arthritis also produces inflammation of the lungs, heart, eyes and the skin. The causes of rheumatoid arthritis are autoimmune disorder, viral and genetic.

The typical symptoms are swelling, redness, warmth, pain and stiffness of the affected joint early in the morning. These symptoms usually last for more than an hour. As the disease progresses, erosion and destruction of the joint surface impairs movement and produces deformity. The common deformities are ulnar deviation, Z-thumb, boutonniere and swan neck. Ulnar deviation also known as ulnar drift involves swelling of the metacarpophalengeal (big knuckle at the base of the finger) joint causing the fingers to become displaced toward the little finger. Z-thumb deformity involves the fixed flexion and subluxation at the metacarpophalengeal joint such that there is shifting of the wrist towards the thumb and the fingers incline toward the little finger. Boutonniere involves deformity of the fingers and toes, where the joint nearest the knuckle is bent toward the palm while the farthest joint is bent back farther. Swan neck involves deformity of the finger in which the joint closer to the fingertip is bent toward the palm and the nearer joint to the palm is bent away. Aside from swelling and deformity of the joints, fever, fatigue, weakness, chest pain, breathing difficulty and anorexia (loss of appetite) occur. The presence of a lump known as rheumatoid nodule in the skin is also apparent.

Diagnosis is done through x-rays and blood tests for rheumatoid factor in the blood. Laboratory results indicate elevated WBC, sedimentation rate and rheumatoid factor. The presence of rheumatoid factor confirms the diagnosis as well the x-ray results.

Treatment consists of analgesic, anti-inflammatory drugs and DMARD (disease modifying anti-rheumatic drugs). Methotrexate and sulfasalazine are examples of DMARD. Biological agents such as interleukin blockers may be prescribed. Synovectomy (removal of synovial fluid) is performed during the early stages of the disease. Exercise programs are recommended to maintain fitness and optimal functioning. Symptomatic management includes bed rest during episodes of exacerbation, intake of 1,500 ml of fluid to prevent renal calculi and application of heat and cold packs. The application of heat reduces stiffness or spasm and cold reduces swelling and pain. The treatment of rheumatoid arthritis involves the entire healthcare team and the cooperation of the client. Home care and management is most effective when client is actively participating in selfcare.

Nursing Care Plan 1

Nursing Diagnosis # 1

Chronic pain related to the degeneration of joints.

Assessment

*Verbal complaints related to painful joints, facial grimaces, withdrawal, restlessness, irritability, refusal to cooperate in activities and decrease in the ability to perform ADL (activities of daily living).
*Assess the client's description of pain in regards to location, intensity and trigger factors.
*Identify trigger factors such as activities and events that precipitate pain.
*Assess the client's method of relieving pain.
*Determine the client's emotional responses and coping abilities in relation to pain.

Expected Outcome/Goal

The client will verbalize reduction and relief of pain after the application of pain reducing interventions.

Therapeutic Interventions

Develop a regimen for relieving pain.
*Instruct the client to change position frequently and move body parts constantly to enable circulation around the affected area.
*Instruct the client to apply hot packs to reduce muscle spasm and stiffness, and apply wet packs to reduce swelling and painful sensation.
*Instruct the client to take prescribed analgesics and antiinflammatory medication such as NSAIDs (non-steroidal anti-inflammatory drugs, e,g. ibuprofen; salicylates, e.g. aspirin), corticosteroid (e.g. cortisone) and centrally acting muscle relaxants (e.g. cyclobenzaprine).
*Explain side effects and adverse effects that can occur when taking such medications.
*Instruct the client to take adequate rest periods between activities to enable the body in coping with pain and discomfort.
*Instruct the client to use assistive devices such as walker and cane if necessary to reduce stress on the joints and assist in ambulation.
*Instruct the client to medicate before an activity or exercise to enable participation and less perception about pain.

Evaluation

The client's verbalized reduction of pain using the pain scale, and stated degree of comfort with medication and pain relieving interventions.

Nursing Care Plan 2

Nursing Diagnosis # 2

Impaired physical mobility related to restricted joint movement.

Assessment

*Client is reluctant to move, has decreased strength, has limited ROM and refuses to perform ADL.
*Assess the client's ROM (range of motion) to determine degree of progressive loss.
*Assess the client's posture and gait to determine gait stability and movement.
*Assess the client's ability to perform ADL and if assisted devices are utilized.
*Determine the client's ability to adapt to physical disability such as in using assistance from significant other or assistive devices.

Expected Outcome/Goal

The client will demonstrate the ability to move or perform ADLs with comfort after health education, supervision and assistance.

Therapeutic Interventions

Develop an activity regimen that focuses on accomplishing ADLs.
*Instruct the client on how to perform isometric and ROM (active and passive) exercises to promote circulation, mobility, strength, coordination and prevent the occurrence of contracture.
*Instruct the client to rest between activities to conserve energy and reduce stressing the joints.
*Encourage the client to use assistive devices as necessary to avoid stressing the joints.
*Discuss and suggest strategies related to transferring, getting out of bed, arising from chairs and picking objects up in ways to to conserve energy and reduce undue pressure to the joints.
*Discuss environmental barriers to mobility such as long flights of stairs.
*Coordinate with a physical therapist and physician for an exercise program suitable for the client.
*Provide written materials related to the client's condition to assist in understanding the disease process and its symptoms, and in clarifying some misconceptions
*Provide a list of support group that may provide additional information and resources to the client.

Evaluation

The client demonstrated the ability to perform ADLs comfortably and efficiently.

Nursing Care Plan 3

Nursing Diagnosis # 3

Fatigue related to the disease process.

Assessment

*Client verbalizes lack of energy, sleepiness and exhaustion.
*Client appears weakened and without interest.
*Assess for decreased functional capacity.
*Determine the client's sleeping pattern.
*Determine if client has co-morbid condition such as anemia.
*Assess the client's gait and psychomotor coordination.
*Determine if client is compliant to prescribed mobility guidelines.

ExpectedOutcome/Goal
The client will verbalize higher level of energy after therapeutic interventions.

Therapeutic Interventions

*Acquire vital signs and coordinate CBC (complete blood count) to determine the existence of anemia.
*Provide the client with adequate rest periods between activities throughout the day.
*Provide health teaching regarding principles of energy conservation.
*Encourage the client to pace activities such as alternating rest and activity.
*Encourage the client to organize activities throughout the day.
*Provide health teaching and demonstration regarding the use of assistive devices to reduce pressure on the inflamed joints.
*Provide and demonstrate gentle range of motion exercises.
*Review mobility guidelines.
*Encourage the client to participate in rehabilitation and physical therapy.
*Teach and demonstrate progressive muscle relaxation exercises to the client.
*Coordinate with physical therapist and rehabilitation specialist as needed.
*Coordinate with a sleep hygienist if needed.

Evaluation

The client verbalized higher level of energy after therapeutic interventions.

Chapter 3 Nursing Care Plans for Alzheimer's Disease

Aging or senescence is a path for everybody. It is not a choice but the direction of life. Diseases accompany aging. The most common disease condition that many associate with aging is dementia of the Alzheimer's type. A diagnosis of Alzheimer's disease almost always invokes uncertainty and doom. This is primarily because Alzheimer's disease has no cure and it is degenerative affecting memory and cognition. A client diagnosed with this condition is extremely challenged and a major burden is imposed on caregivers and family members during the late stages of the disease.

Alzheimer's Disease is a disease where there is mental deterioration due to the presence of tangles and plaques in the brain. It is classified as the most common dementia affecting older adults. It is a chronic and progressive disease with no cure at this point in time. It is believed to be a result of the infiltration of neurofibrillary tangles and amyloid plaques. Neurofibrillary tangles are destabilized structures of the nerve cells while amyloid plaques are clumps of protein peptides. The commonly noted areas of mental deterioration or difficulty are judgment, orientation, confabulation, affect and memory. Judgment is impaired causing socially inappropriate behavior. Orientation is affected causing confusion and perceptual disturbances such as illusions and hallucinations. Affect is affected causing unstable emotions such as outbursts of anger, withdrawal, tearfulness, quarrelsome and mood swings. Memory is impaired causing circumstantial and tangential speaking patterns.

The symptoms in dementia are manifested according to stages. There are 4 stages of Alzheimer's disease; pre-dementia, early, moderate and advance. Pre-dementia is characterized by subtle problems in orientation, attentiveness, planning, abstract thinking, flexibility and semantic memory. This is also known as the stage of mild cognitive impairment. The early stage of this disease is characterized by deterioration in memory and retention, profound confusion, apraxia, agnosia, shrinking vocabulary and decrease in word fluency. Apraxia is inability to execute a learned purposeful movement while agnosia is the inability to recognize objects, persons, sound, shapes and smell. The moderate stage of this disease is characterized by loss of reading and writing skills, impairment of long term memory, behavioral problems becoming prevalent such as wandering and irritability, urinary incontinence and inability to perform activities of daily living. The advanced stage of this disease is characterized by total and complete dependence, loss of verbal language ability and inability to feed oneself.

Diagnosis is made from observations, history, MRI (magnetic resonance imaging) and CT (computed tomography) scans. There is no cure for Alzheimer's disease. Drugs such as acetylcholinesterase inhibitors are prescribed in an attempt to slow the deterioration of the neurotransmitter acetylcholine. This neurotransmitter is responsible for transmitting signals in the brain. Aricept and exelon are acetylcholinesterase inhibitors. Psychosocial interventions such as behavioral therapy are utilized to manage problematic behaviors. Caregiving is an essential part of the intervention to assist the person in coping with the disease.

Nursing Care Plan # 1

Nursing Diagnosis # 1

Self-care Deficit: Bathing, Grooming, Feeding related to cognitive impairment

Assessment

*Client forgets to change clothes, bath, self-groom, perform hygiene, self-feed and self-care.
*Client refuses to perform and cooperate in self-care and feeding.
*Client is confused, disoriented and resistant.
*Assess cognitive difficulties in performing self care and feeding.
*Assess for level of independence and degree of assistance in performing self-care and feeding.

Expected Outcome/Goal

The client participates in performing self-care and feeding after supervision and redirection.

Therapeutic Interventions

Develop a regimen for self-care
*Instruct the caregiver to assist with self-care activities such as bathing, hygiene, grooming and feeding.
*Instruct the caregiver to provide simple and easy-to-do activities on a daily basis such as hair combing and teeth brushing.
*Instruct the caregiver to provide simple food choices and assistance in self-feeding.
*Instruct the caregiver to follow an established daily routine for self-care and feeding.
*Instruct the caregiver to provide the client sufficient time to finish an activity in a quiet environment.
*Instruct the caregiver to encourage the client to perform self-care and feeding as independently as possible.
*Instruct the caregiver to use distraction techniques, simplify tasks, speak calmly and offer praise and encouragement when client refuses to participate in self-care and feeding.

Evaluation

The client participated in performing self-care and feeding.

Nursing Care Plan # 2

Nursing Diagnosis # 2

Stress Urinary Incontinence related to degenerative changes in the muscles of the urinary bladder.

Assessment

*Client complains of physiologic factors such as distended bladder, urinary urgency and frequency.
*Client verbalizes leakage of urine during activities and during coughing and sneezing.
*Client is confused, disorientated and agitated.
*Assess the genitourinary integrity of the client such as the perineal skin and presence of pelvic relaxation such as sagging.
*Assess the behavioral symptoms that may cause urinary difficulties such as confusion, disorientation and agitation.

Expected Outcome/Goal

The client maintains continent of urine after therapeutic interventions.

Therapeutic Interventions

Develop a voiding regimen:
*Instruct the caregiver to provide and encourage adequate hydration to the client and reduce fluid intake after 6 in the evening.
*Instruct the caregiver to assist the client to the bathroom as needed and report symptoms of urinary incontinence, UTI (urinary tract infection) and retention.
*Instruct the caregiver to encourage the client to use urinal and bedside commode at night.
*Instruct the caregiver to assist the client in perineal hygiene, maintaining continent pads, diaper and keeping dry.
*Instruct the caregiver to assist the client to perform Kegel exercises to strengthen the muscles of the urinary bladder.
*Instruct the caregiver to fill a chart stating the times of voiding and occurrences of leakage or incontinence.
*Instruct the caregiver to encourage the client to comply with the bladder retraining program.
*Instruct the caregiver to provide the client with the prescribed medications such as oxybutynin or urecholine as scheduled.

Evaluation

The client was able to maintain urinary continence after therapeutic interventions.

Nursing Care Plan # 3

Nursing Diagnosis # 3

Risk for Injury related to cognitive impairment.

Assessment

*Client verbalizes confusion and disorientation about the house environment.
*Client wanders and gets lost inside the house.
*Assess the client's ability to recognize dangers and hazardous situations such as smoke and fire.
*Assess the client's frequency of confusion and disorientation about home environment.
*Assess the caregiver or family member's understanding of the client's need and degree of cognitive deficits.
*Assess the caregiver and family member's resources and ability to cope with the client's cognitive decline.

Expected Outcome/Goal

The caregiver and family member provide a safe environment for the client.

Therapeutic Interventions

*Conduct a home assessment to determine risks and hazards.
*Involve the family members and caregiver in home care planning and management.
*Provide instruction about removing hazards and risks in the house such as access to matches, tangled electrical cords and back doors.
*Provide suggestions for safety and wandering such as identification bracelet, security devices and emergency system.
*Instruct the caregiver and family members about supervising and monitoring for the client's safety.
*Encourage caregiver and family member to perform a daily supervised walking program to decrease episodes of wandering.
*Provide resources such as support groups and written materials related to home caring for a cognitively impaired person.

Evaluation

The caregiver and family member provided a safe environment for the client after therapeutic interventions.

Chapter 4 Nursing Care Plans for Diabetes Mellitus

The diagnosis of diabetes mellitus to a client imposes a challenge in terms of understanding the disease process as well complying to the treatment regimen. Diabetes is a chronic condition that does not have a cure due to its complicated nature. Research and thorough investigation have provided healthcare professionals with treatment modalities to promote quality of life for a diabetic individual.

Diabetes Mellitus (DM) is a condition where there are metabolic diseases affecting the levels of glucose (sugar) in the blood. The glucose in the blood originated from the intake of carbohydrates from food sources. Carbohydrates are digested in the intestines and passed to the liver for conversion into glucose. After conversion, glucose is transported into the blood stream to be utilized as energy by the body.

In order for glucose to enter the cells, it needs the hormone insulin that is produced by the beta cells of the islets of Langerhans in the pancreas. There are 3 types of DM; type 1, type 2 and gestational. Type 1 diabetes is known as IDDM (insulin dependent diabetes mellitus) or juvenile diabetes. It is characterized by the deficient or absent production of insulin by the pancreas. It commonly arises during ages 12 and 14 up to 19. Type 2 diabetes is NIDDM (non-insulin dependent diabetes mellitus); it is also known as adult onset diabetes. It is characterized by insulin resistance and a relatively low level of insulin production. Insulin resistance involves the inability of the insulin receptors and the cells in general to facilitate the entry of glucose into the cell. It results in an excessive concentration of glucose outside the cells. Gestational diabetes is characterized by transient DM during pregnancy. It is believed that the HPL (human placental lactogen) hormone interferes with the utilization of insulin in the cells resulting in insulin resistance during pregnancy.

Prediabetes is a condition where the blood glucose of a person is high but falls short of the diagnosis criteria for type 2 DM. It is believed that many years of prediabetes eventually result in type 2 DM. The causes of DM are autoimmune disorder for type 1 DM while genetic defects (mutation), infection, pancreatic defect (cancer), drugs (glucocorticoid) and body disorders (Cushing's syndrome) are precursors for type 2 DM.

The lcak of glucose in the cells and excessive concentration in the blood gives rise to symptoms such as polyuria (excessive urination), polydipsia (excessive thirst) and polyphagia (hunger). Polyuria occurs when elevated glucose levels exceed the renal (kidney) threshold for reabsorption of glucose, which results in its escape in the urine causing glucosuria (glucose in the urine). The effect of glucosuria is osmotic diuresis as manifested by polyuria. Osmotic diuresis occurs because of glucose molecules that can not be reabsorbed in the tubules of the kidney. Glucose attracts water preventing its reabsorption (osmotic pressure) in the kidney tubules, and it is eventually excreted as urine. When there is excessive urination, dehydration and electrolyte depletion (sodium and potassium) occurs. Dehydration stimulates thirst as a compensatory mechanism resulting to polydipsia. It also causes weakness and headache due to insufficient water and electrolytes.

Polyphagia (hunger) occurs because the nerve receptors in the cells transmit messages to the brain saying they need glucose and hence more calories and carbohydrates. The brain interprets food as the solution for the hungry cell leading to polyphagia.

The complications of untreated DM are retinopathy, foot ulcers, neuropathy, nephropathy, and cardiovascular disease. Diabetic retinopathy involves the destruction of blood vessels in the eye resulting in vision problems. Diabetic foot ulcers, also known as foot gangrene involves the narrowing and destruction of blood vessels in the feet and legs resulting in the ulceration and death of tissue. It may require amputation. Diabetic neuropathy is the irritation of the nerves in the lower extremities giving rise variously to numbness, pain and tingling sensations and functional weakness. Diabetic nephropathy is the narrowing and destruction of blood vessels in the kidney resulting in scaring of kidney tissues and eventually kidney failure. Cardiovascular diseases in DM are due to narrowing and destruction of the arteries eventually resulting in heart problems including heart attack and stroke.

Diabetic emergencies include ketoacidosis and HONK (hyperosmolar nonketotic). Diabetic ketoacidosis is the result of overproduction of ketones from the liver. Ketones are compound substances that are products of fat metabolism. Fat is metabolized and converted to energy in the absence of glucose inside the cells. Diabetic ketoacidosis gives rise to acetone breath, Kussmaul breathing (rapid deep breathing), abdominal pain, altered state of consciousness, nausea and vomiting. HONK is also known as HHS (hyperosmolar hyperglycemic state). Polyuria results in water depletion and higher levels of blood glucose that eventually results in HONK. The characteristic symptoms of HONK are severe dehydration due to elevated osmolarity (relative concentration of solute), weakness, polydipsia, lethargy and coma.

Diagnosis of DM is done with OGTT (oral glucose tolerance test), FBS (fasting blood sugar), postprandial glucose test and glycosylated hemoglobin (hemoglobin A1c or HbA1c). OGTT is a procedure of drinking 75 grams of glucose and measuring blood glucose every 30 minutes or at different intervals. FBS is a procedure of measuring blood glucose 12 hours after eating. Postprandial glucose test is a procedure of measuring blood glucose 2 hours after eating. Currently the acceptable range for blood glucose is 60 to 120 mg/dl of blood glucose. HbA1c is a procedure of analyzing the blood for hemoglobin A1 in the laboratory produced by the average level of glood glucose over the previous three months. The current acceptable range for HbA1c is 4 to 5.9%. It is done twice a year for people who have stable glycemic control and quarterly for those who are not controlling their glycemic level appropriately.

Treatments for Type 1 DM are daily injections of either fast acting (lispro insulin that works within 5 to 15 minutes and remains active 3 to 4 hours), intermediate acting (NPH insulin that works 1 to 3 hours and remains active 16 to 24 hours) or long acting insulin (glargine that works within 1 to 2 hours and remains active for about 24 hours). The treatment for type 2 DM consist of oral hypoglycemic drugs such as metformin, glyburide, glypizide, tolbutamide, troglitazone and chlorpropamide. Hypoglycemia (excessively low level of blood glucose) occurs due to over-intake of insulin or oral hypoglycemic agents.

Foot care is essential to prevent foot gangrene in the presence of diabetic neuropathy which may leave the client unable to feel foot infections and injuries. Proper diet is recommended consisting of low fat, salt and cholesterol and control of carbohydrate intake. An exercise regimen is also recommended because it lowers glucose levels through increasing cellular insulin sensitivity after exercise. Weight reduction is highly recommended for obese people. Management of hypertension and an elevated cholesterol level are also a part of treatment.

Nursing Care Plan # 1

Nursing Diagnosis # 1

Altered Nutrition: Inconsistent with Body Requirements related to the inability of the cells to metabolize glucose.

Assessment

*Client complains of frequent urination, thirst and hunger
*Assess for the current weight and weight history to determine weight fluctuation.
*Assess the client's current nutritional intake and food preferences.
*Identify current diagnosis related to the type of diabetes and if there are complications that exist.
*Assess blood glucose level and blood glucose history.
*Assess for signs of diabetic complication.
*Assess if client is on diabetic medication and the degree of compliance.
*Assess the client's ability to monitor and perform blood glucose testing on a regular basis.

Expected Outcome/Goal

The client maintains adequate nutritional intake as evidenced by resolution of complains, maintaining blood glucose levels within normal limits and achieving an appropriate body weight

Therapeutic Interventions

*Provide instructions and health teaching about insulin injections or intake of oral hypoglycemics as prescribed by the physician.
*Demonstrate the proper technique in insulin administration.
Instruct the client to perform blood glucose testing on a daily basis and write results in a chart.
*Demonstrate the process of blood testing using a glucose home testing kit for monitoring daily level of blood glucose.
*Instruct the client to report any signs and symptoms of diabetic complications such as paresthesia of the foot and blurring of vision.
*Provide written materials about food nutrients and appropriate caloric intake.
*Coordinate with a dietician or a nutritionist to create a diet regimen.
*Encourage the client to include exercise as part of the current lifestyle.

Evaluation

The client maintained adequate nutritional intake as evidenced by resolution of complains, maintaining blood glucose levels within normal limits and achieving an appropriate body weight.

Nursing Care Plan # 2

Nursing Diagnosis # 2

Risk for Ineffective Management of Therapeutic Regimen related to the complicated treatment method for controlling diabetes and its complication.

Assessment

*Client verbalizes confusion and misunderstanding about the treatment regimen.
*Assess the client's knowledge about diabetes, the prescribed medication, blood glucose monitoring, diet plan, exercise program and lifestyle modification.
*Assess the client's physical and mental ability in self-care.
*Assess the client's motivation and willingness to learn about diabetic management and the treatment regimen.

Expected Outcome/Goal

The client demonstrates understanding of and compliance to the treatment regimen.

Therapeutic Interventions

*Discuss diabetes, it's symptoms, complications, diagnosis and treatment.
*Review the treatment regimen and management in regards to medication, blood glucose monitoring, diet plan, exercise program and lifestyle modification.
*Demonstrate the proper technique in insulin administration if there is prescription of insulin injections.
*Demonstrate the process of blood testing using a glucose home testing kit for monitoring daily level of blood glucose.
*Instruct the client to report any signs and symptoms of diabetic complications such as paresthesia of the foot and blurring of vision.
*Provide written materials and educational resources related to diabetes and its treatment regimen.
*Provide emergency phone numbers to include the client's existing emergency referral system.
*Instruct the client about the importance of self-care and safety.
*Reinforce the need and importance of regular follow-up care and check up.

Evaluation

The client demonstrated understanding and compliance to the treatment regimen.

Nursing Care Plan # 3

Nursing Diagnosis # 3

Risk for Ineffective Individual Coping related to the course of treatment.

Assessment

*Client verbalizes indecisiveness, inability to sleep, depression and inability to cope with the treatment regimen.
*Client appears irritable, angry, regressive, resistant and non-compliant to the treatment regimen.
*Assess for existing coping abilities.
*Assess the client's support system and resources.
*Assess the client's understanding of the treatment regimen.
*Assess for factors such as stressors that impair the coping abilities of the client.

Expected Outcome/Goal

The client is able to demonstrate effective coping strategies as evidenced by compliance to the treatment regimen and identification of stressors.

Therapeutic Interventions

*Review the treatment regimen in regards to medication, blood glucose monitoring, diet plans, exercise and lifestyle modification.
*Allow the client to identify difficulty and stressors in adherence to the treatment regimen.
*Encourage the client to verbalize feelings about the disease process and treatment regimen.
*Provide assistance in determining what part of the treatment regimen needs support or modification.
*Encourage client to set goals and praise for the accomplished ones.
*Encourage the client to engage in satisfying and successful activities related to the treatment regimen.
*Provide list of resources and encourage the client to use existing resources.
*Coordinate with a counselor for psychological counseling if needed.
*Encourage client to maintain regular follow-up care.

Evaluation

The client demonstrated effective coping strategies as evidenced by compliance to the treatment regimen and identification of stressors.

Chapter 5 Nursing Care Plans for Hypertension

Elevated blood pressure always identifies hypertension. This is primarily due to its disease process. For some clients, this is a difficult challenge specially since hypertension is mostly asymptomatic and commonly diagnosed during a doctor's visit. Hypertension is a condition where there is elevated blood pressure in the arteries. The current range of blood pressure considered acceptable is 90 to 119 mmhg (millimeters per mercury) systolic pressure and 60 to 79 mmhg diastolic pressure. Systolic pressure is the pressure during contraction of the heart while diastolic pressure is the pressure when the heart is resting between beats. The types of hypertension are primary and secondary. Primary hypertension is not caused by a medical condition while secondary hypertension is due to an underlying medical condition. Hypertension in general is caused by vasoconstriction (narrowing of the blood vessels), excessive salt intake, smoking and medical conditions.

Diagnosis is done by measurement of blood pressure using a sphygmomanometer. Treatment consists of antihypertensive medications; diuretics, beta blockers, calcium channel blockers, ACE (angiotensin converting enzyme) inhibitors, vasodilators and alpha blockers. Diuretics such as furosemide increase the elimination of salt and water. Beta blockers such as atenolol interfere with nerve receptors in the heart causing it to beat less forcefully. Calcium channel blockers such as nifedipine reduce the ability of the arterial walls to contract. ACE inhibitors such as captopril inhibit the activity of the ACE in converting vasoconstrictors (enzymes that constrict the blood vessel) like angiotensin 1 to angiotensin 2. Vasodilators such as hydralazine relax and dilate the arterial walls. Alpha blockers such as doxazosin interfere with impulses that make the arterial wall constrict. Lifestyle modifications such as limited sodium intake, smoking cessation, active lifestyle and weight reduction, are also an integral part of treating hypertension. The complications of untreated blood pressure are stroke and myocardial infarction (heart attack).

Hypertensive crisis is the late stage of hypertension wherein symptoms are evident and severe causing damage to one or more organs in the body. The systolic pressure is greater than or equal to 180 mmhg and the diastolic pressure is greater than or equal to 120 mmhg. There are two known types of hypertensive crisis: malignant hypertension and hypertensive urgency.

Malignant hypertension is also known as hypertensive emergency. The symptoms are severe and intolerable headache, bilateral papilledema (swelling of optic discs of both eyes), retinal hemorrhage (bleeding in the retina), vomiting, hematuria (blood in the urine), dyspnea (shortness of breath), epistaxis (nose bleeding), severe symptoms of anxiety, chest pain and seizures among others. Hypertensive urgency does not have severe symptoms that indicate organ damage but can become malignant if not attended or treated within 24 – 48 hours. The typical symptoms are headache and epistaxis. The immediate treatment for a malignant hypertension is an intravenous sodium nitroprusside injection. This medication will lower the blood pressure through its nitric oxide compound by relaxing the smooth muscles of the blood vessels and reducing peripheral resistance. It reduces the preload and afterload of the heart. If this drug is not available, clonidine and captopril can be used.

Nursing Care Plan # 1

Nursing Diagnosis # 1

Deficient Knowledge related to lack of information about hypertension and it's treatment.

Assessment

*Client verbalizes misconceptions and lack of knowledge about hypertension and its treatment.
*Assess the client's current understanding about hypertension.
*Assess available resources that can help the client such as a BP home monitoring equipment.
*Assess the client's blood pressure and acquire medical history if available.
*Assess the client's lifestyle, food preferences and dietary habits.

Expected Outcome/Goal

The client verbalizes understanding about hypertension and its treatment.

Therapeutic Interventions

*Provide health teaching regarding hypertension, it's types, causes, risk factors, signs, symptoms, diagnosis and treatment.
*Encourage client to ask questions and clarify misconceptions.
*Demonstrate the appropriate technique in taking blood pressure using the BP home monitoring equipment.
*Discuss the results of blood pressure monitoring regarding acceptable levels and hypertensive crisis.
*Provide the client with written materials about hypertension and its treatment.
*Coordinate with a dietitian or nutritionist regarding diet plans and weight loss program if needed.
*Coordinate with a counselor regarding smoking or alcoholism if needed.
*Suggest aerobic exercises if the client is able and refer to physician for a suitable exercise program if needed.
*Provide the client with community resources and support group possibilities.

Evaluation

The client verbalized understanding about hypertension and its treatment.

Nursing Care Plan # 2

Nursing Diagnosis # 2

Risk for Ineffective Management of Therapeutic Regimen related to the complicated treatment method for controlling hypertension and its complication.

Assessment

*Client verbalizes non-compliance with the prescribed medication, diet plan, exercise program and lifestyle modification of the treatment regimen.
*Assess the client's health values and belief system.
*Assess the client's understanding regarding hypertension and its treatment.
*Assess the client's noncompliant behavior.
*Assess the factors or stressors that affect the client's compliance to the treatment regimen.

Expected Outcome/Goal

The client verbalizes a system for taking medication and following the DASH (dietary approaches to stop hypertension) diet plan and exercise program.

Therapeutic Interventions

*Review the disease process and its complications.
*Review the goal of therapeutic regimen, the medications, diet plan, exercise program and lifestyle modification.
*Demonstrate the correct technique in taking blood pressure and interpreting the results.
*Provide health teaching regarding the medications and their side effects.
*Discuss the DASH diet plan emphasizing nutrient intake and its effect on weight loss and over all well-being of the client.
*Discuss the exercise program and its long-term benefits.
*Discuss smoking cessation and other lifestyle modification for the client's benefit.
*Assist the client in developing a system for taking medications, exercising, quitting smoking and eating DASH diet.
*Provide written materials and resources related to the treatment regimen.

Evaluation

The client verbalized a system for taking medication and following the DASH diet plan and exercise program.

Nursing Care Plan # 3

Nursing Diagnosis # 3

Ineffective Tissue Perfusion: Cardiopulmonary related to uncontrolled hypertension.

Assessment

*Client verbalizes difficulty of breathing, palpitation, lightheadedness and coughing.
*Assess for signs and symptoms of hypertensive crisis such as tachycardia, tachypnea, crackles, hypoxia, edema, dyspnea and cough.
*Assess the client's understanding about the treatment regimen for hypertension.
*Assess for factors or stressors that affects the client's compliance to the treatment regimen.
*Assess any existing co morbid conditions.
*Assess the client's referral and support system.

Expected Outcome/Goal

The client will be able to maintain blood pressure within the acceptable range after therapeutic interventions.

Therapeutic Interventions

*Monitor vital signs and note changes in the blood pressure and pulses before and after the administration of prescribed medications.
*Auscultate for lung sounds and note the presence of crackles.
*Administer a fast acting antihypertensive such as nifedipine or sodium nitroprusside to enable vasodilation.
*Administer other antihypertensive medications as prescribed.
*Position the client in semi-Fowler's position to reduce occurrence of intracranial pressure.
*Maintain the client on complete bedrest until blood pressure is maintained at an acceptable level.
*Elevate legs if there is presence of edema to promote venous return and decrease swelling.
*Turn the client every 1 to 2 hours as needed and assist with ambulation if tolerated.
*Provide written information and discuss treatment regimen depending on client's cognitive abilities.
*Provide emergency numbers and encourage the client to report signs and symptoms related to hypertensive crisis.

Evaluation

The client maintained blood pressure within the acceptable range after therapeutic interventions.

Chapter 6 Nursing Care Plans for AIDS

Human Immunodeficiency Virus (HIV) causes AIDS (Acquired Immune Deficiency Syndrome). During the early stages of infection, HIV is usually prevented from continuously multiplying through a series of antiviral medication. In some instances, a client may not comply with the treatment regimen and HIV infection reaches its full-blown stage known as AIDS. The entire process starting from the moment a client is diagnosed up to diagnosis of AIDS is a big challenge for the client due primarily to the complexity of the disease and the threat of death

AIDS is a disease that involves the final stage of HIV infection. The virus, transmitted through body fluids (blood, semen, vaginal secretions and breast milk), invades and destroys the T4 lymphocyte. HIV is primarily spread through sexual contact, needle sharing and by an infected woman to a newborn infant. The T4 lymphocyte is a WBC that destroys infectious organisms.

The initial infection produces symptoms such as fever, fatigue, sore throat, enlarged lymph nodes, skin rash and other flu like symptoms that last for 1 to 2 weeks. An infected person becomes asymptomatic for 5 to 10 years or more. Fatigue, headache and unexplained weight loss are the usual complaints. As the disease progresses: persistent diarrhea, persistent dry or heavy cough and occurrence of opportunistic infection. During this period of time, the virus multiplies and destroys the T4 lymphocytes. Further destruction of the lymphocytes produces symptoms such as fever, night sweats and diarrhea.

There are a few people who maintain a low or undetectable viral load. They are described as elite controllers and long-term non-progressors. AIDS is considered to develop when the T4 count falls below 200. Opportunistic infections then attack the body causing Kaposi's sarcoma (purplish lesions), yeast infection or candidiasis, pneumococcal pneumonia by Pneumocystis carinii, cytomegalovirus, herpes simplex or zoster, hepatitis C and others.

Diagnosis of AIDS and HIV is done with blood testing to determine T4 count and viral load. ELISA (enzyme linked immunosorbent assay) and Western blot tests are the commonly used diagnostic tests for diagnosing this disease. Treatment consists of HAART (highly active antiretroviral therapy), which slows its progression. The HAART are NNRTI, NRTI and PI. NNRTI (non-nucleoside reverse transcriptase) consists of efavirenz (Sustiva), nevirapine (Viramune) and delavirdine (Rescriptor). NNRTI inhibits the movement of the transcriptase enzyme that is needed in the synthesis of the virus. NRTI (nucleoside reverse transcriptase inhibitors) consists of zidovudine (AZT), abacavir (Ziagen), didanosine (Videx) and lamivudine (Epivir). NRTI inhibits the chain reaction in the viral replication. PI (protease inhibitor) consists of ritonavir (Norvir), nelfinavir (Viracept), atazanavir (Reyataz), darunavir (Prezista), tipranavir (Aptivus) and fosampenavir (Lexiva). PI prevents viral replication by binding to viral protease and blocking protein precursors that facilitate production. Antibiotics may be prescribed for infection.

Nursing Care Plan # 1

Nursing Diagnosis # 1

Risk for Infection related to an immunocompromised system.

Assessment

*Client's laboratory result shows decreased CD4 cells, positive HIV antibody and detectable viral load.
*Assess for signs of opportunistic infection such as skin lesions, diarrhea, productive cough and sore throat.
*Assess the client's state of health in relation to vital signs, weight, caloric intake and medical history.
*Assess the client's understanding about AIDS, it's causes, diagnosis, signs, symptoms, treatment and the method for preventing opportunistic infection.
*Assess the client's existing resources and referral system.

Expected Outcome/Goal

The client demonstrates a method for preventing opportunistic infections.

Therapeutic Interventions

*Discuss the disease process, it's causes, diagnoses, signs, symptoms, treatment and opportunistic infections according to client's cognitive abilities.
*Discuss and demonstrate methods of preventing opportunistic infections such as hand washing, avoiding crowded places, bathing, personal hygiene and avoiding cat litter among others.
*Administer the prescribed antiviral medication such as NNRTI (non-nucleoside reverse transcriptase), NRTI (nucleoside reverse transcriptase inhibitors), PI (protease inhibitor) and discuss side effects.
*Provide written materials and community resources that the client can use for support.
*Coordinate with the physician to check for electrolyte values if needed.
*Coordinate with dietitian for diet plan if needed.
*Suggest aerobic exercises such as walking to suit the client's ability and refer to physician for an exercise program.
*Encourage the client to consistently do follow-up care, maintain communication with healthcare providers and report signs or symptoms of opportunistic infection and provide access numbers as necessary.

Evaluation

The client demonstrated a method for preventing opportunistic infections.

Nursing Care Plan # 2

Nursing Diagnosis # 2

Ineffective Individual Coping related to diagnosis of disease.

Assessment

*Client verbalizes inability to make decisions, experiences insomnia, depression, headache, lack of appetite and inability to ask for help.
*Client appears irritable, angry, hostile, powerless and defensive.
*Assess for the client's perception of diagnosis.
*Assess the client's current understanding about the disease process and it's treatment.
*Assess the client's support system.
*Determine if there is suicidal ideation.

Expected Outcome/Goal

The client identifies coping strategies and appropriate resources to use in coping with the diagnosis.

Therapeutic Interventions

*Discuss and provide written materials about AIDS, it's causes, diagnosis, signs, symptoms and treatment according to client's cognitive abilities and emotional tone.
*Allow client to verbalize feelings about the diagnosis.
*Allow client to ask questions and clarify misunderstanding.
*Provide information related to the current needs and desires of the client.
*Provide resources such as support groups appropriate for the client's condition.
*Encourage the client to identify effective coping strategies such as meditation, compliance with medications, social networking and craftsmanship.
*Encourage the client to engage in self-care and report any opportunistic infection to healthcare providers immediately as it appears.
*Support client's decision in a non-judgmental way and praise accomplishments.
*Coordinate with a counselor or a therapist as needed.
*Coordinate with a case manager or a social worker as needed
*Coordinate with hospice care if needed.

Evaluation

The client identified coping strategies and appropriate resources to use in coping with the diagnosis.

Nursing Care Plan # 3

Nursing Diagnosis # 3

Imbalanced Nutrition: less than body requirements related to loss of appetite.

Assessment

*Client verbalizes loss of appetite and weight loss.
*Client appears thin and underweight.
*Assess the client's weight, caloric intake and BMI (body mass index).
*Assess the client's coexisting condition and medications that affects the appetite of the client.
*Assess for an opportunistic infection that affects the appetite of the client such as oral candidiasis that can cause dysphagia.
*Assess the client's feelings regarding the disease process.

Expected Outcome/Goal

The client regains normal weight and does not incur further weight loss.

Therapeutic Interventions

*Discuss and provide written materials about nutrients, caloric intake and dietary supplements according to the client's cognitive abilities.
*Develop a meal plan according to the client's preferences considering nutrient values or caloric intake and in coordination with a nutritionist.
*Assist with meal preparation if needed.
*Administer emetics before eating if nausea and vomiting occurs.
*Administer prescribed antiviral medication and explain those that cause loss of appetite.
*Administer food supplements prescribed by the physician.
*Administer prescribed medication for oral candidiasis to eliminate dysphagia.
*Administer prescribed medications against opportunistic infections that occur in the gastrointestinal tract and other parts of the body.
*Suggest aerobic exercises which reduces fatigue and encourage appetite according to client's abilities and in coordination with the physician.
*Coordinate with a dietitian or a nutritionist as needed.
*Coordinate with a counselor or therapist if needed.
*Provide resources and community support for the client.

Evaluation

The client regained normal weight and does not incur further weight loss.

Chapter 7 Nursing Care Plans for Pneumonia

The respiratory tract is vulnerable to infection primarily because of its ability to inhale air and its particles. Though there are filters in the upper respiratory tract and WBC (white blood cells) that fights infection, these are not always sufficient to protect an individual. Certain foreign entities such as bacteria and virus are strong enough to cause pneumonia. The diagnosis of pneumonia imposes a threat to a client primarily because it affects respiration.

Pneumonia is a condition where there is an inflammation of the lung due to an infection. It affects the air sacs of the lung. Pneumonia can be caused by a bacterium, virus, parasite or a fungus. Hence, the type of pneumonia varies according to the causative agent. Pneumonia is transferred primarily by droplets and direct contact. Certain factors such as upper respiratory infection, excessive alcohol ingestion, depressed CNS (central nervous system), heart failure, COPD (chronic obstructive pulmonary disease), endotracheal intubation and postoperative effects of anesthesia can cause pneumonia.

The typical symptoms are productive cough, fever and chills, shortness of breath, chest pain upon inhalation, fatigue and rapid heart rate. Symptoms can vary according to the type of pneumonia. Clients at risk for developing pneumonia include those who are bedridden, immobile, immunocompromised and hospitalized. Elderly and neonates are also at high risks.

Pneumonia is further classified according to its causative agents such as gram positive pneumonia, gram negative pneumonia, anaerobic bacterial pneumonia, mycoplasma pneumonia, viral pneumonia and protozoan pneumonia. Gram positive pneumonias are usually caused by community acquired pneumococcal, staphylococcal and streptococcal bacteria. Gram negative pneumonias are caused by hospital acquired Klebsiella pneumonia, Pseudomonas pneumonia, Influenza pneumonia and Legionnaire's disease. Anaerobic bacterial pneumonias are usually acquired through aspiration. Viral pneumonia is usually caused by influenza virus. Pneumonia is also classified according to area affected such as lobar, bronchial and lobular

Chest x-ray and a sputum specimen are used to confirm the diagnosis. Treatment will be in accord with the causative agent. An antibiotic is prescribed for bacterial pneumonia. An anti-fungal such as amphoterecin B is prescribed for fungal pneumonia. An antiviral such as acyclovir is prescribed for a viral pneumonia. Analgesic is taken for pain. Oxygen is administered through the nose in some cases. Liquefying secretions and postural drainage are also done to clear the airways. Nursing and medical interventions include IPPB (intermittent positive pressure breathing), incentive spirometry, chest physiotherapy, adequate rest periods, suctioning and diet plans are used.

Nursing Care Plan # 1

Nursing Diagnosis # 1

Impaired Gas Exchange related to the disease related changes in the alveolar capillary membrane.

Assessment

*Client verbalizes difficulty in breathing, confusion and weakness.
*Client appeared cyanotic, restless, tachypneic, disoriented and has tachycardia.
*Client's laboratory result shows decreased PaO_2 and increased $PaCO_2$.
*Assess the respiratory rate, pattern and use of accessory muscles.
*Assess for signs of impending respiratory failure.
*Assess and monitor the vital signs.
*Assess for increasing mental changes, restlessness and weakness or activity intolerance.

Expected Outcome/Goal

The client maintains normal respiratory rate after therapeutic interventions.

Therapeutic Interventions

*Monitor respirations, vital signs and signs of hypoxia.
*Maintain humidified oxygen administration as ordered.
*Position client at semi-Fowler if confined in bed to promote comfort and ventilation.
*Assist client to perform the deep breathing technique and controlled coughing by having the client inhale deeply and hold the breathe for several seconds and cough two or three times with open mouth as tolerated by the client.
*Monitor the oxygen saturation using pulse oximetry while waiting for the blood gas result.
*Auscultate the breath sounds every 1 to 2 hours and note for the presence of crackles and wheezes that can exacerbate the presence of hypoxia.
*Monitor the client's behavioral and mental changes such as lethargy or somnolence that implies severe impairment in gas exchange.
*Assist client to ambulate or exercise if tolerated.
*Turn the client's position every 2 hours to increase oxygenation.
*Assist the client with small frequent meals as tolerated to maintain caloric intake.
*Coordinate with respiratory therapist if needed.
*Prepare the client for intubation or mechanical ventilation if disease condition worsens.

Evaluation

The client maintained normal respiratory rate after therapeutic interventions.

Nursing Care Plan # 2

Nursing Diagnosis # 2

Ineffective Airway Clearance related to presence of excessive respiratory secretions.

Assessment

*Client verbalizes difficulty in breathing and productive cough.
*Assess for abnormal lung sounds such as rhonchi and bronchial sounds.
*Assess for the use of accessory muscles of respiration.
*Assess respiratory status and vital signs.
*Assess the characteristics of sputum and changes that occur.
*Assess for client's coughing and its effectiveness.

Expected Outcome/Goal

The client maintains a patent airway after therapeutic interventions.

Therapeutic Interventions

*Monitor the client's respiratory rate, vital signs and auscultate the breath sounds every 1 to 2 hours to determine presence of coarse crackles and abnormal lung sounds.
*Monitor the blood gas values and oxygen saturation to determine status of oxygenation.
*Position the client in semi-Fowler's if confined in bed to promote lung expansion.
*Assist client to perform the deep breathing technique and controlled coughing by having the client inhale deeply and holding the breathe for several seconds and cough two or three times with open mouth as tolerated by the client.
*Encourage and assist the client in using an incentive spirometer to prevent lung collapse and facilitate movement of secretions.
*Perform suctioning and clearing of secretions as ordered.
*Provide oral care as necessary.
*Encourage ambulation and exercises as tolerated by the client.
*Encourage adequate hydration and fluid intake of 2,500 ml as needed to help move secretions and prevent dehydration.
*Administer prescribed medication such as bronchodilators and inhaled corticosteroid, and watch for adverse effects.
*Perform postural drainage, percussion and vibration interventions if ordered by the physician.
*Coordinate with a respiratory therapist as needed.

Evaluation

The client maintained a patent airway after therapeutic interventions.

Nursing Care Plan # 3

Nursing Diagnosis # 3

Ineffective Health Maintenance related to insufficient knowledge about disease management.

Assessment

*Client verbalizes confusion about treatment methods.
*Assess the client's understanding about pneumonia, it's causes, signs, symptoms, diagnosis and treatment.
*Assess the client's vital signs, existing symptoms and coexisting conditions.
*Assess client's understanding about the treatment regimen.
*Assess the client's existing support and referral system.
*Assess the client's feelings toward the treatment regimen.

Expected Outcome/Goal

The client verbalizes understanding of the disease process and compliance to the treatment regimen.

Therapeutic Interventions

*Review and discuss pneumonia, its causes, signs, symptoms, diagnosis and treatment.
*Encourage client to verbalize feelings regarding the treatment regimen.
*Teach client how to deep breathe and cough and their importance.
*Administer prescribed antibiotics and analgesic and teach client about their effects on the body.
*Perform postural drainage and teach incentive spirometry as prescribed.
*Assist client in prescribed exercises and explain their importance.
*Teach the client about preventive techniques to prevent exacerbation and occurrence of cross infection.
*Teach the client about the importance of adequate hydration and to increase fluid intake to facilitate movement of respiratory secretion.
*Provide written materials about pneumonia and resource materials to provide support to the client.

Evaluation

The client verbalized understanding of the disease process and compliance to the treatment regimen.

References

I would like to express my gratitude to:

Dr. Lee Robbins for his support in writing this book.

Anatomy and Physiology, Wiley and Sons, New Jersey, 2007
Fundamentals of Nursing 7th Edition, Mosby, Canada, 2009
Medical – Surgical Nursing 4th Edition, Prentice Hall, New Jersey, 2008
Nursing Assistants, Mosby, Philadelphia, 2004
Pathophysiology of Disease 2nd Edition, Appleton and Lange, 1997
Pharmacology in Nursing 21st Edition, Mosby, Missouri 2001
The Johns Hopkins Consumer Guide to Medical Tests, Medletter Associates Inc, New York, 2001
Wikipidea Free Internet Dictionary

Connect with me online :

Facebook: http://www.facebook.com/solomon.barroa
Twitter: https://twitter.com/solomonbarroa
Amazon: amazon.com/author/solomonbarroa
LinkedIn: http://www.linkedin.com/in/solomonbarroa

Index

ACE, 23
acetylcholine, 13
acetylcholinesterase inhibitors, 13
adequate hydration, 15, 33, 34
ADL, 10, 11
agnosia, 13
AIDS, 1, 27, 28, 29
Alpha blockers, 23
Altered Nutrition, 20
Alzheimer's disease, 1, 13
ambulation, 10, 26, 33
amyloid plaques, 13
analgesics, 8, 10
anorexia, 9
antihypertensive, 23, 26
anti-inflammatory drugs, 9
Apraxia, 13
Aricept, 13
Arthritis, 8
Arthroplasty, 8
Arthroscopy, 8
assessment, 4, 7, 16
asymptomatic, 23, 27
atenolol, 23
autoimmune disorder, 9
bacterial pneumonia, 31
Beta blockers, 23
bladder retraining, 15
blood glucose, 17, 18, 20, 21, 22
blood pressure, 23, 24, 25, 26
blood testing, 20, 21, 27
blood vessels, 18, 23
Bouchard's nodes, 8
Boutonniere, 9
bronchodilators, 33
Calcium channel blockers, 23
caloric intake, 20, 28, 30, 32
captopril, 23
carbohydrates, 17
caregiver, 14, 15, 16
cartilage, 8, 9
chest pain, 9, 23, 31

Chronic pain, 10
clonidine, 23
cognitively impaired, 16
cold packs, 9
communication, 7, 28
compliance, 20, 21, 22, 25, 26, 29, 34
confusion, 13, 15, 16, 21, 32, 34
contractures, 8
cope, 16, 22
coping abilities, 10, 22
coping strategies, 22, 29
coughing, 15, 26, 32, 33
counselor, 22, 24, 29, 30
crackles, 26, 32, 33
crepitus, 8
DASH, 25
data, 7
data gathering, 7
deep breathe technique, 32, 33
Deficient knowledge, 24
deformity, 8, 9
degenerative changes, 8, 15
dehydration, 17, 18, 33
demonstrate, 11, 12, 22, 28
Diabetes Mellitus, 1, 17
Diabetic foot ulcer, 18
Diabetic ketoacidosis, 18
diabetic management, 21
Diabetic neuropathy, 18
Diabetic retinopathy, 18
Diagnosing, 7
diarrhea, 27, 28
diastolic pressure, 23
diet plan, 21, 25, 28
dietitian, 24, 28, 30
difficulty in breathing, 32, 33
difficulty of breathing, 26
disease management, 34
disease process, 7, 11, 12, 17, 22, 23, 25, 28, 29, 30, 34
Diuretics, 23

DMARD (disease modifying anti-rheumatic drugs), 9
doxazosin, 23
dysphagia, 30
dyspnea, 23, 26
electrolytes, 17
ELISA, 27
energy, 11, 12, 17, 18
epistaxis, 23
Evaluating, 7
exelon, 13
exercise program, 11, 21, 24, 25, 28
exercises, 8, 11, 12, 24, 28, 30, 33, 34
feeding, 14
feelings, 22, 29, 30, 34
fever, 8, 9, 27, 31
fibrous ankylosis, 9
fluid intake, 15, 33, 34
follow-up care, 21, 22, 28
frequent urination, 20
Fundamentals of Nursing, 35
furosemide, 23
glucose, 17, 18, 19, 20, 21
glucosuria, 17
HAART, 27
hazards, 16
HbA1c, 18
headache, 17, 23, 27, 29
Heberden's nodes, 8
hematuria, 23
HIV, 27, 28
HONK, 18
hydralazine, 23
Hypertension, 23
Hypertensive crisis, 23
hypertensive emergency, 23
Hypoglycemia, 18
hypoxia, 26, 32
IDDM, 17
Imbalanced Nutrition, 30
immunocompromised, 28, 31
Impaired Gas Exchange, 32
Implementing, 7
incentive spirometer, 33
Independent nursing actions, 7
Ineffective Airway Clearance, 33

Ineffective Health Maintenance, 34
Ineffective Individual Coping, 29
Ineffective Tissue Perfusion, 26
inflammation, 8, 9, 31
insulin, 17, 18, 20, 21
interdependent nursing action, 7
intermediate acting, 18
IPPB, 31
joint stiffness, 8
Kegel exercises, 15
lifestyle modification, 21, 22, 25
long acting insulin, 18
loss of appetite, 9, 30
lung sounds, 26, 33
Malignant hypertension, 23
mechanical ventilation, 32
medication, 10, 20, 21, 22, 23, 25, 27, 28, 30, 33
memory, 13
mental deterioration, 13
metacarpophalengeal, 9
metformin, 18
mobility, 11, 12
muscle spasm, 8, 10
neurofibrillary tangles, 13
NIDDM, 17
nifedipine, 23, 26
NNRTI, 27, 28
NRTI, 27, 28
NSAIDs (nonsteroidal antiinflammatory drugs, 10
nursing care plan, 4, 7, 8
nursing diagnosis, 4, 7
nursing process, 4, 7
nutrients, 20, 30
nutritionist, 20, 24, 30
Objective data, 7
OGTT, 18
opportunistic infection, 27, 28, 30
oral hypoglycemics, 20
orientation, 13
osmotic pressure, 17
osseus ankylosis, 9
Osteoarthritis, 8
osteophytes, 8
oxygenation, 32, 33

PaCO2, 32
PaO2, 32
patent airway, 33
physical therapist, 11, 12
physician, 7, 11, 20, 24, 28, 30, 33
PI, 27, 28
Planning, 7
Pneumonia, 1, 31
polydipsia, 17, 18
polyphagia, 17
polyuria, 17
postural drainage, 31, 33, 34
pre-dementia, 13
Prediabetes, 17
Primary hypertension, 23
problem, 4, 7
productive cough, 28, 31, 33
protozoan pneumonia, 31
pulse oximetry, 32
redirection, 14
resources, 11, 16, 21, 22, 24, 25, 28, 29, 30
respiratory therapist, 32, 33
rest periods, 10, 12, 31
Rheumatoid Arthritis, 9
rheumatoid factor, 9
Risk for Ineffective Individual Coping, 22
Risk for Ineffective Management of Therapeutic Regimen, 21, 25
Risk for Infection, 28
Risk for Injury, 16
ROM, 11
secondary hypertension, 23
secretions, 27, 31, 33
self care, 9, 14, 21, 29
Self-care Deficit, 14
semi-Fowler's, 26, 33

smoking cessation, 23, 25
sodium nitroprusside, 23, 26
sphygmomanometer, 23
Stress Urinary Incontinence, 15
Subjective data, 7
support system, 22, 26, 29
Swan neck, 9
swelling, 8, 9, 10, 23, 26
Synovectomy, 9
synovial joints, 9
Synovitis, 9
synovium, 9
systolic pressure, 23
T4 lymphocyte, 27
therapeutic interventions, 12, 15, 16, 26, 32, 33
transferring, 11
treatment, 9, 17, 18, 21, 22, 23, 24, 25, 26, 27, 28, 29, 34
treatment regimen, 17, 21, 22, 25, 26, 27, 34
Type 1 diabetes, 17
Type 2 diabetes, 17
Ulnar deviation, 9
understanding, 11, 16, 17, 21, 22, 24, 25, 26, 28, 29, 34
urinary continence, 15
urinary urgency, 15
vasoconstriction, 23
vasoconstrictors, 23
Venipuncture, 1
viral pneumonia, 31
vital signs, 12, 26, 28, 32, 33, 34
wandering, 13, 16
weight, 8, 20, 23, 24, 25, 28, 30
weight loss, 8, 24, 25, 30
Z-thumb deformity, 9

***Kindly write a review about this book for Amazon or other sites to help other readers that could benefit from this text. Thank you.**

And please feel free to browse my other books @ Amazon.com

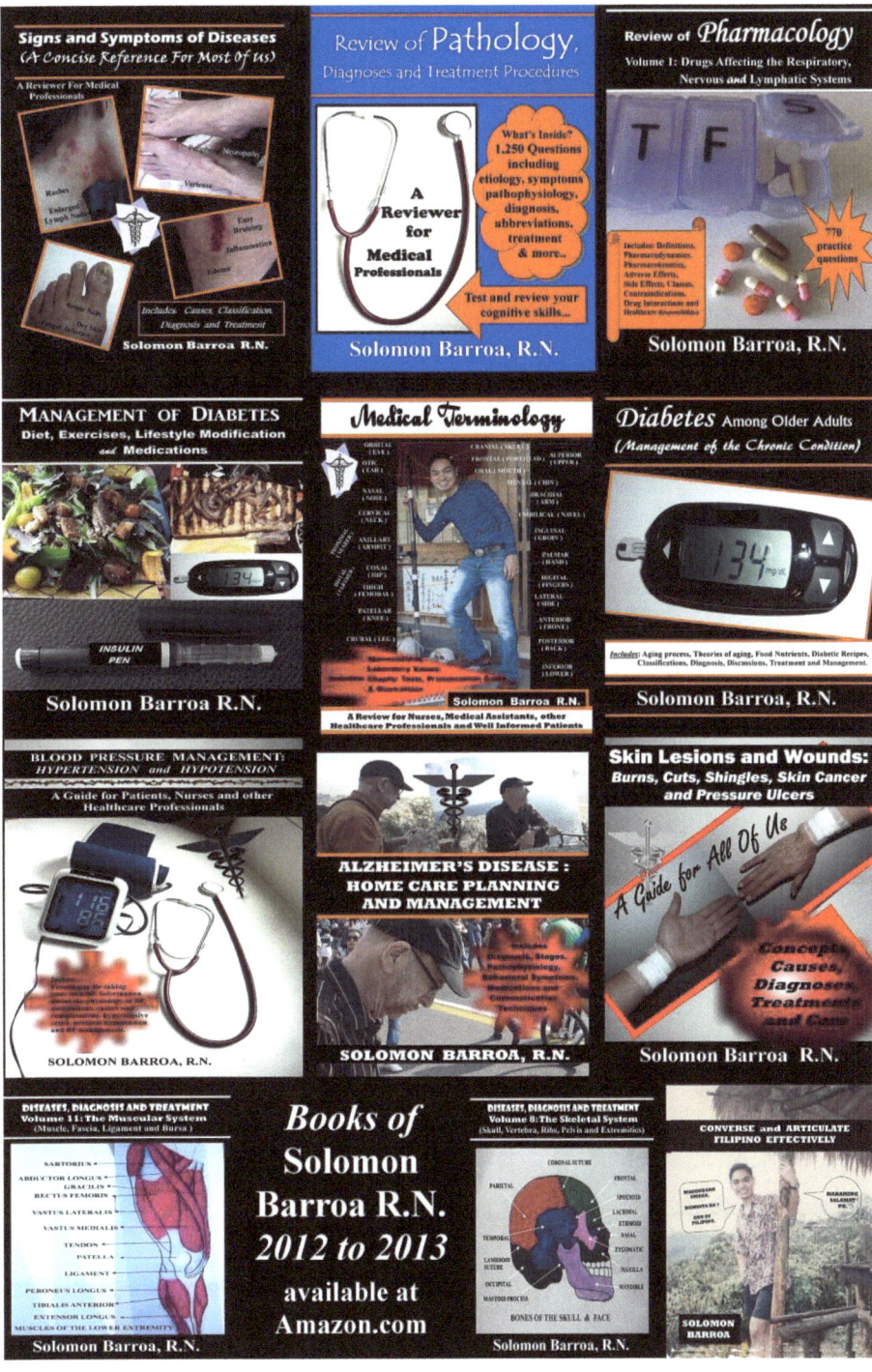

www.ingramcontent.com/pod-product-compliance
Lightning Source LLC
Chambersburg PA
CBHW040754200526
45159CB00025B/2100